RIA KANG

10-Minutes A Day Skincare Hacks For Beginners

A Simple Step-By-Step Guide To Radiant Skin With Essential Ingredients

Contents

1

Introduction

Taking care of your health is a must these days. People invest a lot of time and money into weight-loss medicines, doing workouts, and eating healthy and organic foods. That's for your body as a whole. Now what about your skin? Your physical health is important to your skin health, but there's more than just eating healthy in order for your skin to glow like Rihanna's. That's what we're all here to learn more about. It's skincare.

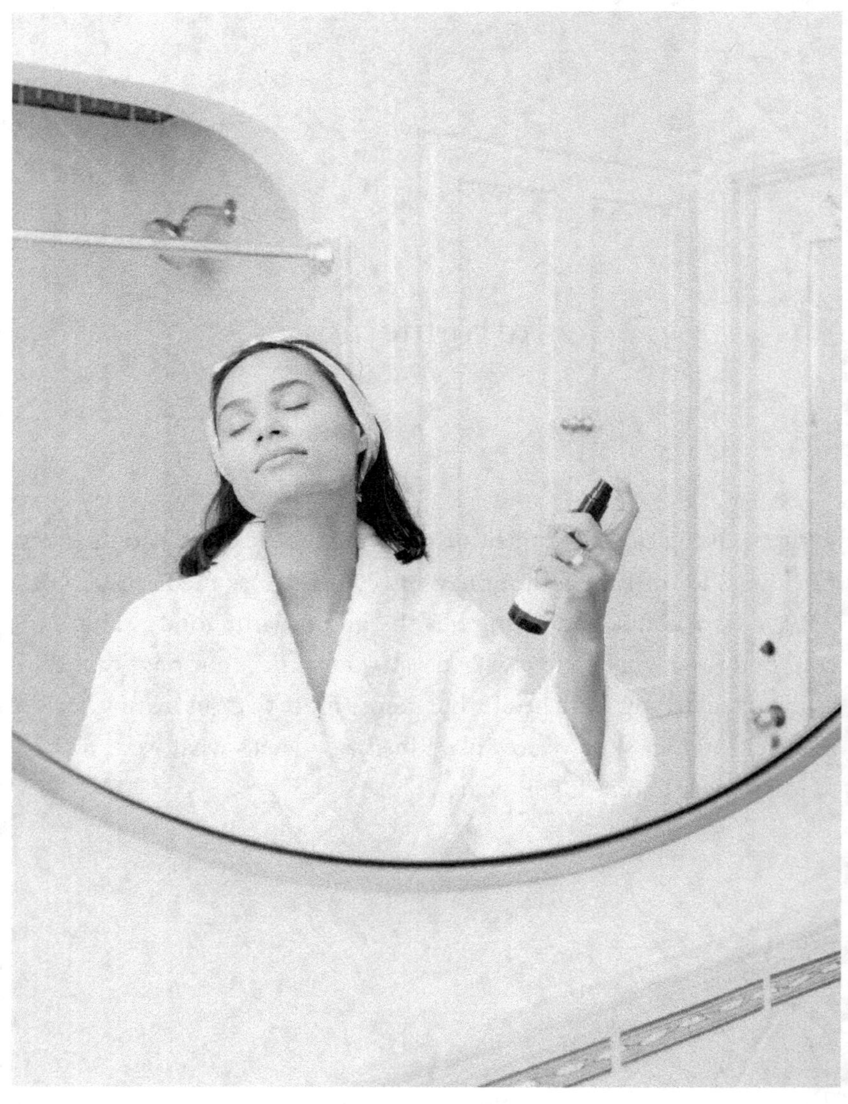

I started skincare routines since I was in elementary school, all thanks to K-Beauty trends that I saw when I was still living in Korea. There were so many beauty brands and shops on the streets, and I remember just buying one of the best sellers without much thought. All I knew was I needed to apply lotion on my face after washing it. Is that the same for some of you? My grandma would wash my face with water and put lotion on, and that was basically it for my childhood's skincare routine. But there is so much more than just putting lotion on your face.

As I grew older and learned from other people, I got to know more about different skin types, skincare products that are available, when and how to use each, etc. The more you learn, the more you realize you don't know much. There were so many layers to explore in order to make your face shinier! This doesn't necessarily mean that taking care of skin is difficult or complicated, though. It was all about finding the right one for me to use and understanding how to use each.

Skincare routines are unique to each one of us. We all have different skin types and complications to consider, and understanding the cause of the skin problems you have can help you tremendously. This book is a short, condensed guide for you to know the basics of the skin, common skin concerns, steps of skincare routines, and healthy habits to kick off your daily skincare routines. Think of this book as your friend who's a skincare enthusiast telling you how to start your skincare journey. Let's get started!

2

Why Is Skincare SO Important?

Before we jump into skincare, let's take a closer look at the skin itself. Your skin basically protects your inner organs from the outside. There are three layers to skin, which are epidermis, dermis, and hypodermis, in the order from outermost to innermost. Epidermis is the ultimate protector of all the layers. It prevents bacteria and other harmful elements from entering our body. Dermis is in the middle and contains collagen, which helps your skin stay firm. This is the thickest of all and where other main components such as hair, oil, and sweat comes from. No wonder why it's so thick! The bottom-most layer, hypodermis, is a bridge between the outer layers and the inner body system such as nerves, muscles, and bones.

Well that's enough for the anatomy lesson. But this will come in handy for later chapters.

So why do we need skincare? There's a common myth about skin, which is that you don't need to really care for your skin until you are older. Let me tell you, no matter how young you are or how you look outside, your skin starts aging at the age of 25, on average. You are lucky if you are still less than 25 and reading this. I was lucky that I knew as an elementary school student that I needed to do some kind of skincare everyday. But don't panic either if you are over 25. You can start taking care of your skin and slow down skin aging from now.

More common myths are like, "we need to wash our face with hot water," "we can use toothpaste to treat a zit faster," and "acne only happens to teens." These are not true! First of all, hot water increases the temperature of your skin which will make your skin dry. I wish I knew this earlier because I enjoy showering with hot water and having a feeling of removing all the grease off my face with hot water. Secondly, toothpastes aren't for your skin but for your teeth. It's common sense people. This is not a DIY treatment for your skin. And acne doesn't care about your age. Teenagers are more likely to experience acne because of hormonal changes, but that doesn't exclude adults from getting acne.

What about habits you are ignorant about, such as sleeping with makeup on OR on the other side of the spectrum you wash your face too often? Makeup containing bacteria from outside needs to be removed before you go to bed because this is when your skin repairs itself. On a similar note, touching your face with your hands that contain millions of bacteria will get you acne. Hands are known for having more bacteria than the toilet in your bathroom. As much as it sounds gross, it is true. So stay away from touching your face with unwashed hands! And if you are washing your face too much, on the other hand, it will only make your face itchy and drier, not necessarily cleaner.

Plus, healthy skin will not only make you look younger but also prevent skin disorders and diseases. The most common ones being acne, hives, spots, etc. Think of skincare as supplements you take for your body health. If your dermis lacks collagen, using skincare products that contain collagen will make your skin more firm. Dull skins can become brighter using vitamin c serum. Just like this, you can find a solution to your skin problems through customizing your skincare steps and using the right products. Prolonged skin conditions can only lead to stress and more severe symptoms, so don't be neglectful about it.

I used to think that my acne would disappear as time went by. But that wasn't the case at all because my bad habits of sleeping late, eating irregularly, wearing make-up for too long until early morning, and most importantly what I used for my skincare didn't change. This has become one of my favorite quotes after learning the hard way: "Expecting difference without changing anything is insanity." I needed to make changes in my life in order to change how I looked. If any of you are thinking similarly to myself in the past, please I advise you not to make the same mistakes I made. Being ignorant of the problem until it gets very severe and now that I'm trying to fix it, it takes a much longer time and effort to get back. Start taking care of your skin today. Or even better, if your skin is still healthy and young, keep it that way!

3

What Is My Skin Type?

There are about 5 different skin types in general: normal, oily, dry, combination, and sensitive. You can also take skin type surveys online that can tell your skin types more in detail.

To figure out your skin type quickly, first look at the amount of oil on your face. If your skin generates a lot of oil throughout the day, you'll more likely have oily skin. It'll be mainly on your T-zone, that is your forehead and nose area, as well as your cheek area. You may easily break out due to clogged pores from oil. On the other hand, if your skin feels rough and tight, and you have fine wrinkles throughout your skin, your skin is closer to a dry type. If neither fits your skin, then you might have normal skin (as normal as it sounds, it's neither oily or dry) or combination skin. Combination skin has both oily parts and dry parts throughout the face. Most combination types will have oily T-zone and normal or dry condition throughout other parts of the face. Last but not least, the sensitive type can apply to any of the above skin types. Whether your skin has a lot of oil or not, it can sensitively react to outside factors, such as dust particles, and have physical symptoms.

There's no one-size-fits-all skin type. Some people may have different combinations of each skin type. It can also change anytime throughout your life, and understanding your skin conditions won't be overnight. My skin was dry when I was young, and now it's oily and more prone to acne and sensitive to dust. It may take some time for you to see the patterns in your skin conditions, but take your time. If you feel like your skin texture has changed or is reacting to different substances, take a skin type test again. It might have changed. Once you have a better understanding of your current skin type, you can now move on to figuring out what the skin concerns you have.

4

Most Common Skin Concerns And Essential Skincare Ingredients You Need

There are a lot of skin conditions that you may face throughout your lifetime. It can change as you move to a new environment, eat different foods, age, etc. Let's talk a little bit about the most common skin concerns and what's causing them to bother us so much. And most importantly, we'll see what are some main ingredients that we can look for when we go out to buy our skincare products!

Acne: One of the most common skin concerns many of us have is acne. Also called pimples or zits. They are from pores that are clogged by oil, dead skin cells (also known as sebum), and bacteria. That's why oily skin types usually have acne as their #1 skin concerns. These clogged pores, if not cleaned and treated regularly, can form into acne which can turn into whiteheads, blackheads, and pimples. Pimples happen when our body's immune system reacts to and fights the bacteria in acne. That's why they cause redness and inflammation.

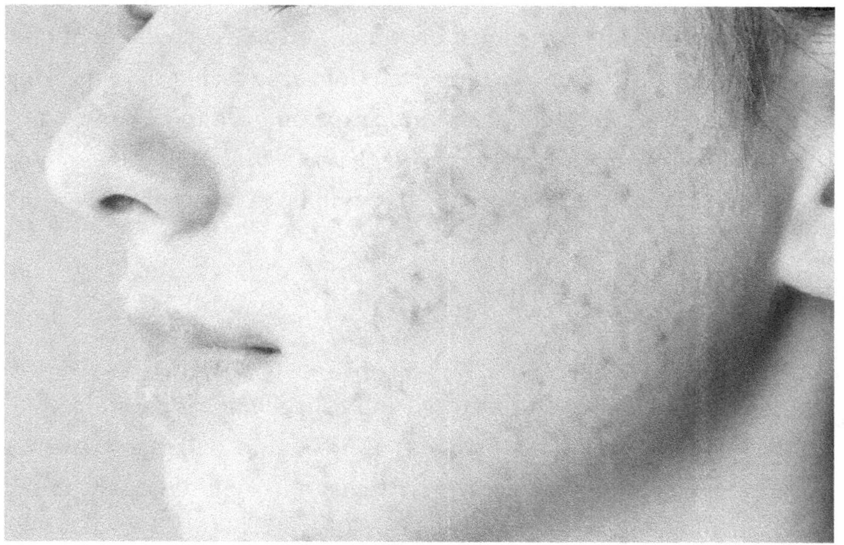

Essential Ingredients:

- **Salicylic Acid or BHA (Beta Hydroxy Acids)** helps reduce redness of the inflamed area and remove dead skin cells. Good for cleansing pores, too. My cleansing routine involves a cleansing oil product with BHA inside which is a perfect combination for deep washing of the pores.
- **Tea Tree** ingredients can reduce inflammation of acne. Its smell may be too strong for some people sensitive to smells of nature or herbs.
- **Panthenol** is a type of Vitamin B and is helpful for decreasing oil production.

Large Pores: When you look at the mirror closely, you may notice small holes throughout your face. The sizes will vary from person to person, but if you can see your pores easily, you may have larger pores which will make your skin look more rough and dehydrated. Your pores can get large due to a lot of sebum excretion, acne that keeps appearing on the same spot, and inelastic skin. Also, you need to be careful not to scrape your acne or blackheads. If they are forcefully removed or squeezed out too hard, you may be left with large pores in those spots.

Essential Ingredients:

- **Retinol** will help remove dead skin cells from the pores and expedite the process of skin cell and collagen production.
- **Peptides or PHA (Poly Hydroxy Acids)** will strengthen your skin barriers and thus enhance the elasticity of it. Peptides can be in the form of collagen.
- All the ingredients that help with acne reduction so the pores won't get larger in the first place!

<u>Spots/Scars:</u> If you have spots and scars from acne or your skin tone is not even, pay attention! There are 2 main scars from acne: Depressed (Atrophic) and Raised (Hypertrophic). To put it simply, depressed scars are from lack of skin cells during the healing process after the acne has been removed, and raised ones are the exact opposite of it - too many skin cells forming while recovering. For the uneven skin tones, it's more likely your skin is experiencing oxidation, where your skin cells are damaged by the free radicals around them.

Essential Ingredients:

- **Vitamin C** is a key helper for brightening dark spots. It's one of the antioxidants which literally means anti-oxidation. This will make the healing process faster.

- **Rosehip Oil** contains Linoleic Acid that increases collagen, thus aids with a proper skin healing process.
- **Salicylic Acid and Retinol** also help with acne scar reduction. AHA, another kind of Hydroxy Acids similar to BHA, is also helpful for cleansing of the pores, which reduces the scarring.
- **SUNSCREEN!** A lot of discoloration is due to excess sunlight absorbed into the dermis layers of the skin. We'll cover the application of sunscreen in the later chapter.

<u>Aging</u>: This is not only for people who are physically old. If your face has fine lines and wrinkles, dark spots, and is even sagging or dehydrating as if it's going to crack? You are experiencing aging of the skin. It can show on all parts of your body but if it especially shows on your face or your neck, it makes you look older than you are, sadly. But skincare products that have the following ingredients can help slow down the process of aging.

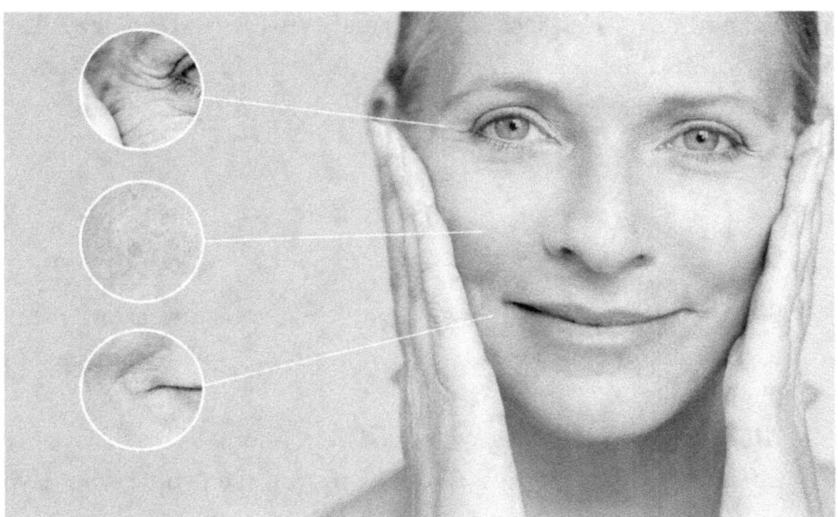

Essential Ingredients:

- **Retinol**, as it promotes the collagen production, can reduce dehydration and sagging (inelasticity) of your skin.
- **Panthenol** is an anti-aging ingredient as it hydrates, smooths your skin and helps strengthen your skin barriers.
- **Madecassoside** is a type of plant extract that enhances the skin's hydration and can act as an antioxidant like Vitamin C to fight against the skin damage and repair the skin barriers. I have been using toner pads that are concentrated with madecassoside extracts for about 8 months now, and it's been super helpful in moisturizing and healing damages from continuous acne breakouts.

<u>Eczema</u>: People experiencing rashes especially during the cold seasons will more likely have eczema. This is caused by your top-most layer of your skin (epidermis, going back to the 1st chapter) being broken and exposing the bottom layers to outside factors. Eczema on the face may often appear on creases, such as eyelids and even ears and feel itchy. The key to treating this is moisturizing as far as treatment through skincare. Severe eczema may need to be treated through prescribed medicine or cream so consult with your doctor.

Essential Ingredients:

- **Shea Butter** is well-known for its rich moisturization effect. It contains linoleic acid that eczema-prone skins don't have in themselves.
- **Aloe Vera** can help heal wounded skin and is used for its anti-inflammatory properties. This is why you see people who have sunburns apply aloe vera all over their body. Likewise, aloe helps

suppress the redness from eczema.

- **Petrolatum (petroleum jelly)**, as oily as it sounds, keeps the water inside the skin barriers to prevent dryness. The most common one you see in the stores is called Vaseline (I remember my grandma used to put this on my face every night..)
- **Niacinamide** is part of the Vitamin B family and rebuilds the damaged skin cells and barriers.

5

10-Minute Skincare Daily Routines

Now that we have more background knowledge about our skin, we'll look at how to incorporate skincare routines in our daily life.

Disclaimer, if you are saying you don't have enough time for adding another set of routines in your schedule, that's just an excuse. Everyone of you has 10 minutes, 20 minutes max, in a day that you can spare from your Netflix time or being on your phone. And it's more soothing and refreshing to be involved in this routine especially before you go to bed. Imagine you went to work for 8 hours or hung out with your friends until night, came back home and slept with oil produced all day long and bacteria from outside on your face. I can get grosser but I won't. This is why I highly encourage you all to practice this routine at least once a day, if not twice a day, to avoid all the skin concerns we've talked about before.

#1. Cleansing

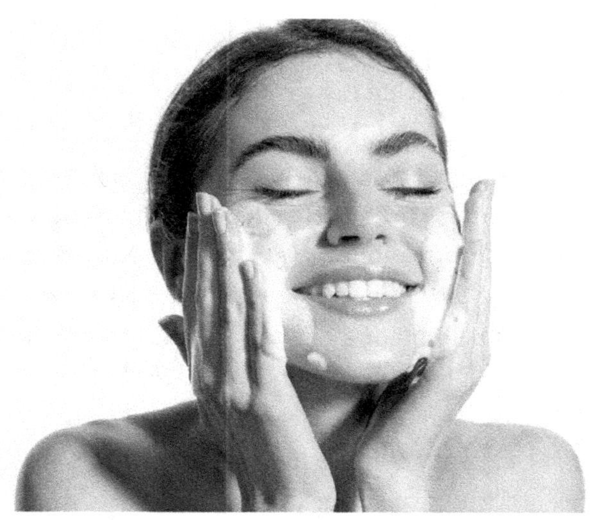

First and foremost, you need to wash your face before applying any of the skincare products. I break my skincare routine into two different times: morning and night. You may wonder why you would need to wash your face in the morning when you stayed indoors all night and didn't even put makeup on. Like I mentioned before, your skin repairs during the night when you are asleep, during which it regenerates skin cells and heals the damaged cells. This means that your skin surface may have excess amount of skin cells and dead cells, and to not have them clog your pores during the day, you must get rid of them when you wake up.

AND remember to wash your hands before cleansing!

Cleansing products have different types:

- Cleansing Oil: this type is usually recommended for deep cleansing of the pores, as you roll your fingers with oil on your face for about 1-2 minutes, your sebum and blackheads will dissolve to a certain extent where they get removed. Because it's oil, this wouldn't dry your face during the cleansing process as much as other types do.
- Cleansing Gel: this type requires you to rub your hands together in order to make it into a foam or bubbly form, which then is applied to your face for 30 seconds to 1 minute and washed off.
- Cleansing Foam: this type is already a foam, meaning it reduces the time of the cleanser foaming while getting applied onto your face. That's helpful for dry skin types as they need to spend as little time as possible on cleansing their face. It doesn't mean that you can be sloppy about the cleansing process, but you need to be careful leaving your face too long with the cleanser on or water on which can dry out your face quickly.
- Cleansing Wipes: this type of cleanser can come in handy for traveling as it's in the form of wipes and already has the cleansing components on them. Only thing you need to do is wipe off your face with it, but you need to be careful not to rub your face too hard.
- Cleansing Water: this type is more mild compared to others as it is mainly made of water. You can wash with it like washing with running water or use cotton pads or a cloth to absorb the cleansing water and gently massage the face to cleanse.
- Lip & Eye Remover: this one is made specifically for lip and eye makeup. This remover usually consists of oil solution, which needs to be shaken each time before using. Use cotton pads or a cloth to absorb the remover and put these on top of the applicable parts, leave for 15-30 seconds and gently rub them off. Depending on the thickness of the makeup, you may need to repeat this process until you don't see any residual on the cotton pads.

Each type will have different kinds of products for different types of skin. When you buy one, read the description and find the one that fits your skin type. And please remember to wash your face with warm water, until the cleanser is removed completely. After washing, I recommend not to wipe off the remaining water with a towel or rub it off too hard. There may be bacteria on the towel that's been hanging in the bathroom, so I usually only absorb excess water falling down and try not to touch my face as much as possible.

#2. Exfoliation/Facial Masks

This step may be customized to fit your skin type and routine, meaning that it can be included once or twice a week and skipped for the other days.

Exfoliation is for removing the excess sebum or blackheads, and the products usually come with grainy texture/particles for rubbing off the sebum and blackheads. I would describe it as rubbing sticky sugar against my face, specifically for the product that I'm using. Some may contain more than others, so please see the product descriptions and consult with skincare experts if needed. Also, some cleansers may include exfoliation in themselves, so that can help minimize the steps you need. Lastly, exfoliation shouldn't be included in your routine more than 2 times a week. If you exfoliate everyday, it can damage your epidermis, so be careful not to do this too often or exfoliate too hard.

Facial masks can also be optional for your routine. You can think of it as a bonus for your skincare, where you fill in your needs with extra care. There are many types of face masks, from wash-off clay masks, peel-off masks to sheet masks. And each one of them should fulfill your skin concerns' treatment, such as brightening, hydrating, firming, calming, etc. Usually, wash-off types will take you less time to wait and will require you to wash your face again. Sheet masks will take you more time, depending on each brand and function, and don't require you to wash again. Some sheet masks may have you leave them on for up to 20 minutes, which may sound very long but you can do other stuff while waiting too. I usually lay down on my bed and stretch my legs or watch TV during that time. Facial masks can be customized into your skincare routine, where you do this twice a week, every week, every 2 weeks, and etc.

#3. Toner

If you are skipping step 2, you would apply toner right after you wash your face. Don't take too long to apply the toner, as it will dry out your face quickly. Toner acts as extra cleansing plus a quick hydration before the next step. After you do the step 1, you may still have some makeup, cleanser, and dirt remaining deep inside your pores. You can use the cotton pads to absorb toner and gently rub it against the face.

Some people say this step can be skipped as well, but it is highly encouraged as it gets rid of impurities once more! It will reduce the chance of clogging your pores and getting acne.

Toner will come in liquid most of the time or in the form of pads. Pads are ready-made products where you can use the pads directly. Depending on each product and what ingredients it has, these pads may act as facial masks where you leave the pads on for an extended time for the ingredients to absorb into your face. I personally prefer toner pads because I don't have to buy cotton pads separately for toner and can be a quick alternative for facial masks.

BONUS When you select cotton pads for toner, consider the thickness of each pad and how much liquid it absorbs. If it's too thick or soaks up too much, it will use up a lot of toner quickly and might not be economical. Some pads are designed specifically for toners and are very thin and soft to use. These are recommended for those who'll use them as quick facial masks as well.

#4. Serum

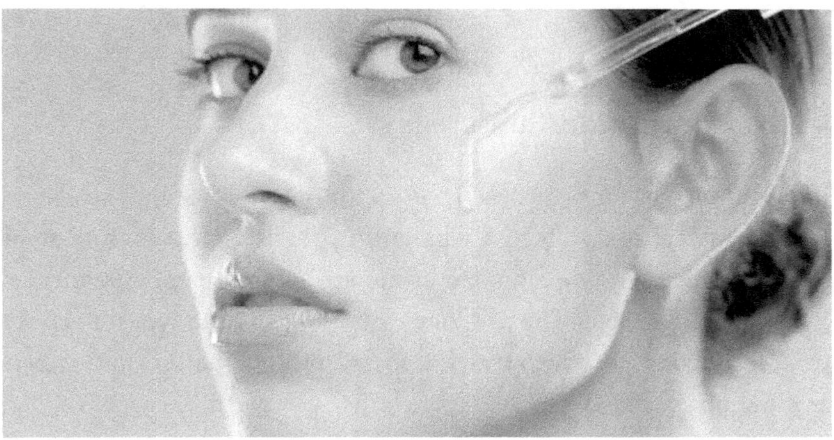

This step is also optional like face masks. Serums are concentrated liquids designed for each specific skin condition. They are similar to face masks in a way but more concentrated. This step comes before the hydration of your skin in order for it to absorb deeply into the dermis layers before the hydrating product blocks it.

They often come in a pipette dropper container, where you can apply or drop onto a specific part of your face. Some products may allow you to mix several amplified solutions with the base serum, so that you can tailor it to your needs. For example, I have dark acne scars in my cheeks, and my face looks dull. I'd mix anti-spot solution and brightening solution to make my own serum which can solve both of my problems!

There are so many serums that can boost skin health, but as much as they are highly concentrated for the skin concerns, they are usually on the pricier end among all the products involved in this routine. So please go through options you have and make a choice according to your needs and circumstances.

#5. Moisturization/Sunscreen

Last but not least, moisturization is up for next. This step is crucial as it's going to act as a protective barrier for your skin after all these steps of caring. These will be named as moisturizing cream, moisturizer, hydrating cream, etc. The products will differ by skin types, so check what it contains and which type it is for. Consult with the beauty expert at the shop if needed.

Also, some moisturizers may contain SPF, or Sun Protection Factor. Going back to our 1st chapter, there are 3 layers of dermis in our skin. And there are 2 types of UV light in sunlight: UVB and UVA. UVB only penetrates into the outermost layer of the skin, epidermis, while UVA can penetrate into the middle layer Dermis. 95% of the sunlight consists of UVA which can kill collagen and cause skin cancer, so it's very important that you find the right sunscreen.

The SPF only tells you how much UVB light is protected with the product. The higher the number of SPF, the more UVB light it protects. SPF 30+ is the minimum you need, and in order for it to protect you from UVA as well, find the one with a broad spectrum. So SPF 30+ or higher with the broad spectrum protection will protect you from both UVA and UVB.

But be aware that no sunscreen can be treated as a complete protection from the sun. It's better to avoid long exposure to sunlight and constantly reapply in order for it to have lasting effect.

You may use regular moisturizer at night, while using the one with SPF during the day. Or you may choose to buy a separate sunscreen to use after the moisturizer before you go outside.

Cost For Skincare Products

So these 5 steps are the basic guideline you can follow to customize your skincare routines. If you are starting off with no skincare experience at all or need to restart with a completely new set of products, here are some general estimates for the cost of each step.

- Cleanser: $15-$40
- Exfoliator: $18-$45
- Facial Masks: $6-$10/sheet for sheet masks OR $30-$60/bottle of wash-off masks
- Toner: $10-$40 for a bottle OR $20-$40 for toner pads (60-70 pads for each)
- Serum: $10-$200
- Moisturizer: $20-$70

- Sunscreen: $20-$50

This is just for your reference to start budgeting, but each product that's designed for different needs will have different prices. It also depends on the size of each product. That's why these ranges are very broad. Do your own research or visit stores to calculate how much you need to make your own skincare set.

I totally understand if you think this is expensive just to make your skin look nicer. I feel that way too because every few months I buy new skincare products. But please keep in mind that this price is not for one time use only. Each bottle of 400-500ml, depending on how many times you do your skincare per day, will last at least for a few months if not the entire year. Exfoliators and facial masks will be used only 1-2 times/week. You won't use more than a pea-size drop for one time application of sunscreen. If you think about one time cost and how long you'll use for each product, it won't be as expensive as you thought it was. Trust me, the investment will be worth it!

6

Additional Habits

Now that you are all set up with your own skincare routine, here are a few more tips to get you started on your skincare journey.

#1. Healthy Diet & Drinking Water

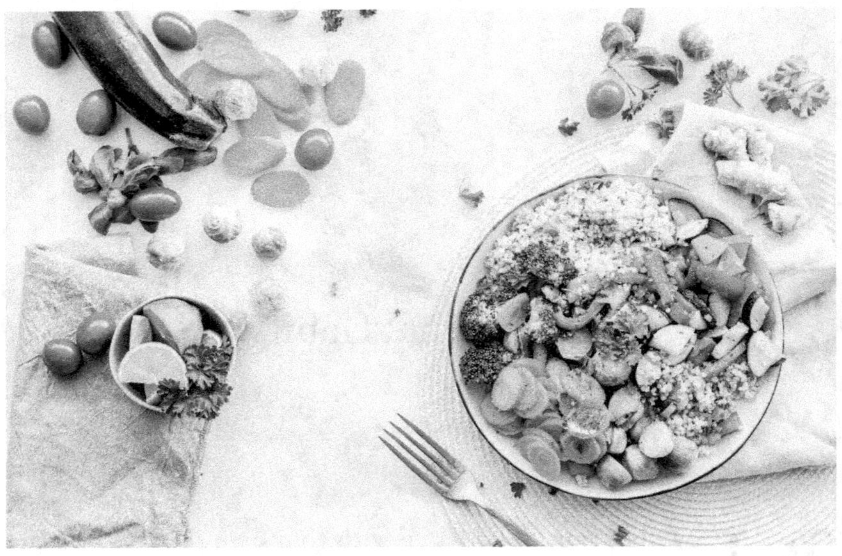

I won't make it another lecture from your mom about eating healthy. But it is true that your diet is another key contributor to your skin health. You can tell if your digestive system is functioning well when you look at your face. Eating a lot of vegetables that contain fiber and drinking a lot of water will make your digestive system healthy and enhance the excretion activity. If not, toxins will appear on your face in the form of acne and pimples. So be sure to consume vegetables regularly and drink water throughout the day, at least 3-4 of 500ml water bottles.

#2. Apply Sunscreen Regularly

I can't stress the importance of sunscreen enough. Please go back to the previous chapter if you need a reminder of why sunscreen is so important. UV lights in the sunlight are detrimental to skin if not protected properly and can ultimately lead to skin diseases such as skin cancer. And make sure you use sunscreen even if it's cloudy. UV lights can go through the clouds even if you can't see them. C'mon, it will only take a minute or so to put sunscreen on your face.

#3. Sleep Well

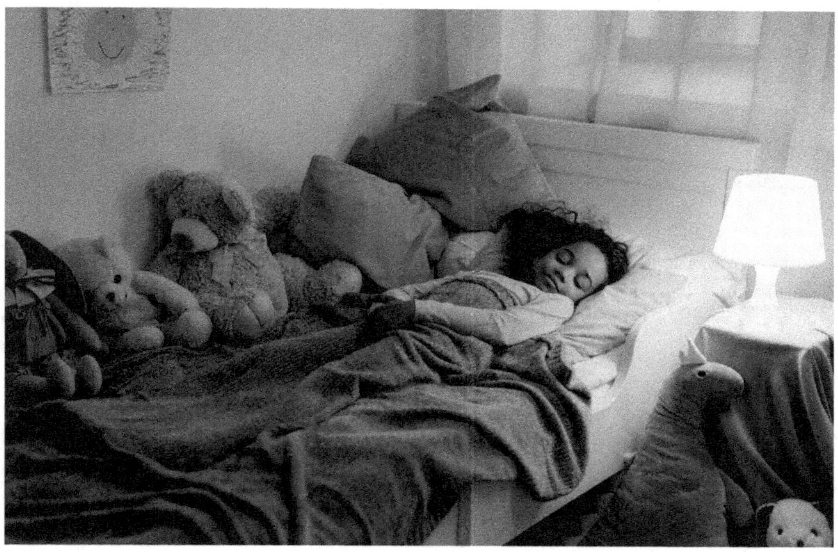

Keeping the regular sleep schedule and not staying up too late will significantly enhance the quality of your skin and body health as a whole. Average amount of sleep that's needed for a person is 7-9 hours per day. Not getting enough sleep can increase the chance of aging, puffy eyes, rough skin surface, and acne production. It's best to start sleeping between the body repair time which is 10pm to 2am, to provide the best condition for the repair to happen. Your health will be revealed through your appearance. Sleep well!

7

Conclusion

This is just the beginning of mastering skincare. Now remember, consistency is the key. Regardless of your age, your skin has been adapted to the current condition and care for an extended time. It will take time and dedication for your skin to adjust to your new routine and for you to see the result of enhanced skin condition. Be patient with yourself and stay committed. I'm on the same boat with you, as I keep trying new products to make my routine better and better. Achieving our dream skin quality is an ongoing pursuit, and there's no turning back. We all are on the path to healthier and brighter skin that is yet to come.

If you like this book, kindly leave a review on Amazon and share your thoughts and routines with others! Best luck to all of you!

8

Resources

- *Your guide to the most common skin concerns - NØIE - NØIE.* (n.d.). NØIE. https://noie.com/skin-concerns
- Professional, C. C. M. (n.d.). *Skin.* Cleveland Clinic. https://my.cle velandclinic.org/health/body/10978-skin
- Norris, P., & Norris, P. (2019, September 18). 50 skin care myths. *Norris Dermatology & Laser Northwest.* https://www.norrisderm.co m/50-skin-care-myths/
- CeraVe. (2023, June 13). What Type of Skin Do I Have? *Cerave.com.* https://www.cerave.com/skin-smarts/skincare-tips-advice/what-skin-type-do-i-have
- *Salicylic acid topical: Uses, side effects, interactions, pictures, warnings & dosing - WebMD.* (n.d.). WebMD. Retrieved March 31, 2024, from https://www.webmd.com/drugs/2/drug-18-193/salicylic-acid-to pical/salicylic-acid-for-acne-topical/details
- *Access anytime anywhere | Cleveland Clinic.* (n.d.). Cleveland Clinic. https://my.clevelandclinic.org/
- Sublime Life. (2020, June 16). 13 powerful ingredients that get rid of stubborn acne scars. *Sublime Life.* https://sublimelife.in/blogs/s

ublime-stories/13-ingredients-tired-and-tested-to-work-on-even-stubborn-acne-scars

- Contreras, L. Y. a. a. G. (2024, February 29). *What are free radicals and how do they affect skin?* ISDIN Blog. https://www.isdin.com/en-US/blog/skincare/your-skin/what-are-free-radicals-how-do-they-affect-skin/
- Moi, C. (2020, February 27). *Why Panthenol (Vitamin B5) is a Skin Saver — Chez Moi De Beaute: 30 Years of Beauty.* Chez Moi De Beaute: 30 Years of Beauty. https://www.chezmoi.com.sg/blog/panthenol
- *Best and Worst cosmetics ingredients for eczema: 6 to love, 4 to leave.* (n.d.). WebMD. https://www.webmd.com/skin-problems-and-treatments/eczema/ss/slideshow-best-and-worst-cosmetic-ingredients-for-eczema
- Alexander, H. (2021, May 28). What does SPF mean? *MD Anderson Cancer Center.* https://www.mdanderson.org/cancerwise/should-you-use-very-high-spf-sunscreen.h00-159460845.html#:~:text=Before%20you%20buy%20sunscreen%2C%20it%27s,you%20from%20getting%20a%20sunburn
- *Makeup, skincare, fragrance, hair & beauty products | Sephora.* (n.d.). Sephora. https://www.sephora.com/